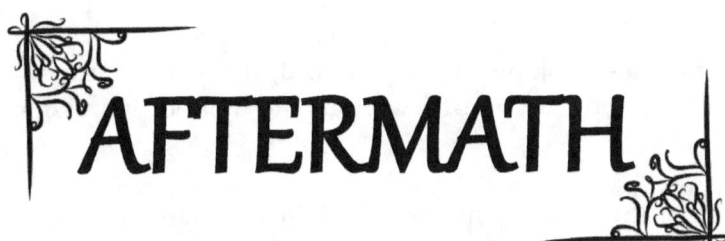

AFTERMATH

The Sequel to Hospital Survival

By

Jay Morrow

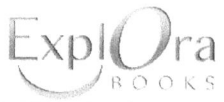

EXPLORA BOOKS
700–838 West Hastings St. Vancouver, BC V6C 0A6
www.explorabooks.com
Phone: (604) 330 6795

No part of this book may be reproduced, stored in a retrieval system, or transmitted by any means without the written permission of the author.

Because of the dynamic nature of the Internet, any web addresses or links contained in this book may have changed since publication and may no longer be valid. The views expressed in this work are solely those of the author and do not necessarily reflect the views of the publisher, and the publisher hereby disclaims any responsibility for them.

ISBN: 978-1-998394-32-6

© 2024 Jay Morrow. All rights reserved

AFTERMATH

A Harrowing Journey of Healing

JAY MORROW

Table of Contents

MY LIFE BECOMES INTERESTING

After surviving my hip infection, as detailed in "Hospital Survival" I developed a reverence for life that I never had before I realized that I should try and enjoy life's experiences while I could. My wife and I love to travel and see/experience new cultures and sights, but I am limited in what I can do. I can't fly for eight hours, stand in lines, and walk unlimited distances. Cruising seemed like a great solution.

As I was sailing on my tenth cruise after my final recovery from my many surgeries, I sat across from a couple who were talking about their trials with an illness where the man had collapsed after a trip to Europe. He had finished a trip to Greece, with an additional trip to Jordan, Israel, and Egypt. Somewhere in Egypt, he contracted an unusual strain of pseudomonas, that had progressed to septicemia by the time they had returned to British Columbia, Canada. His hands and feet were numb because the germ had blocked arteries in both his hands and feet.

They tried to combat it with standard antibiotics, but they proved ineffective against this new strain. They ultimately had to amputate his hands at the wrists and legs at the calf. He had prosthetics for his legs, but his forearms terminated at stumps. Overall, he and his wife's spirits were still excellent. As he described his illness, I waited until he finished, and the conversation had settled into the usual topics of plans for the next port of call and what everyone planned on accomplishing during the day. I looked across at his wife and said: "I can beat that story." She looked incredulous at me and said, "What".

My story began with my hip, which led to my permanent impairment and loss of mobility told in my first story "Hospital Survival", how I had developed a mysterious unknown infection and lost my career. Although this story was told in a previous book, the events were a full five months of torture for me. It led to the loss of half of my femur, and my hipbone, and a full year of life in a wheelchair. I was a cripple, lost my career and it led me to consult, western antibiotics, Chinese herbs, acupuncture, massage therapy, and holistic medicine; looking for a cure.

Every time I visited my orthopedic surgeon, he told me that they couldn't tell if the infection had been cured. My blood chemistry was so screwed up that they could not tell if the infection had passed, and I could not receive a prosthetic hip until I was "infection free". I admit that after this discussion, I broke down and cried in his outer lobby. My wife was there to buck me up, but I could not see how much more I could do to get well.

When I consulted the Chinese doctor, he examined my tongue. He had me stick it out and showed it to me in the mirror. It was black. He said I was very sick, but he thought he could help me. He also grabbed my wrists and evaluated my "CHI". He started a regimen of Chinese herbs and acupuncture that helped immensely. After three months of treatment, my tongue was pink and healthy. I went back to my surgeon for a consultation on a new hip.

The surgeon ran a series of blood tests to see if I was still infected by staph. The results were still completely inconclusive. The surgeon told my family, but not me; that I might still be infectious. He asked if I would consent to an exploratory operation to check on the status of the post that had been inserted in the hip to just hold the muscles in place. He said if everything was fine, I would get a new type of titanium post and a new plastic hip. The operation proceeded and he was shocked to find me infection-free. He then removed the metal post that he had inserted earlier and gave me a titanium split shaft that was inserted into a plastic hip joint. If the operation had shown that I was still infected, he would just seal me up and I would never walk again. Because the infection had gone, I would be in the operating room for 4-5 hours and was in the recovery room quickly with a new prosthetic hip.

I woke up 8 hours later in the recovery room. I was still under the effects of the anesthetic, so I felt wonderful. Three days later, I left the hospital and climbed into our Prius for the trip to the rehab center. I was released to the rehab center to re-learn how to walk. After two weeks in rehab, I was released to go home and continue with rehab on an outpatient basis. I would go to my local rehab gym to work out under a physical therapist three days a week for the next three months.

Once I recovered, my wife decided to finally retire in 2007. She loves to travel and has been to most places in the world. She recently went to Tibet, Nepal, Singapore, and most of Southeast Asia. This was preceded by trips to Peru, Easter Island, Chile, Antarctica, Argentina, and Brazil. I went on none of those trips, simply because my leg won't hold up to her extensive walks, and long-distance airfares.

So now, if she is not going too far on an airplane, I just say when are we going? We have been to the Caribbean, Alaska, Mexico, and the East Coast. We especially like cruising since I can use the workout room and visit some ports where the walking is not extensive or overwhelming. I enjoy it immensely because we are also committed to meeting new people on each cruise. Usually, we ask to sit at a table, without reservations, and ask for open shared seating. This usually means sitting with new people each night and hearing their histories and tales. Invariably, they have some story about a hospital or medical situation. I usually just remain silent unless they ask me about my situation, or why I walk funny. Once I had an opening and began to tell them about my medical history, they listened raptly for the first half an hour. At which point I tell them; I am only a third of the way through my tales of the medical trials and tribulations.

The group on the cruise ship is already astounded about my hip. Their eyes widened as I covered the loss of the hip. But I had to tell them that this was only the beginning of the story. They asked me to continue to tell the remainder of the story. The entire table is already engrossed with the tale as were others in close proximity to our table. After the first story, they all wanted to hear the next segments of the story. I rattled off my complete tale of woe for the next hour.

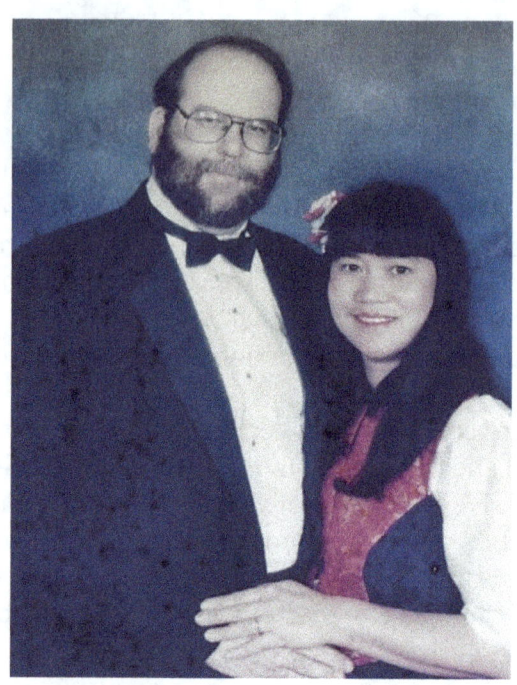

Our first cruise picture

I began my extensive tale of woe that occurred over the next 14 years in total. I had the rapt attention of the people at our table as they strained to hear the details of my journey through various hospitals and operations. Most people became incredibly engrossed by the story and by my wife, who is the heroine of much of the story. My wife usually lets me tell the story, but she would jump in to cover the areas where she was essential to my survival.

There was only once that I curtailed my story at that point. As I was telling of the septicemia portion of my story, a person whose son had died from septicemia had to leave the table since it brought up such negative feelings. I apologized to their friend and asked them to convey my sorrow and to ask for their forgiveness for even bringing the subject up at the dinner table.

ATTITUDE HAS ITS OWN IMPACTS

As I covered in my first book, I had had a major problem with an infection on my hip. After my five months in the hospital, I was a muscle-shriveled mass and overweight. When I was finally released from the hospital, I was still without a fully functioning hip. The hospital had determined that they could not help me become infection-free, so I was released on my recognizance to attempt to get healthy on my own. They released me to a rehabilitation center and I began my recovery. I was still incredibly weak from spending 5 months confined to a bed in the hospital before I was finally released. This may seem irresponsible on my part, but I needed to get away from the hospital and its costs. Since I had been sentenced to 5 months of bedridden pain, my muscles had severely atrophied and the stump ended at the top of the femur, with no hip joint to bear my weight.

I spent several weeks just getting used to the wheelchair. I had a trapeze on the bed that allowed me to transfer my weight from the bed to the wheelchair. I had a bare stump that extended from the half of the remaining femur to the bare remains of my hip socket (or what remained of it). I could not put my full weight on the joint, but if I was careful with a walker, I could (with supervision) walk about 10-15 feet. Afterward, as my arm strength improved, I began to race down the hallways in my wheelchair, check out the dining hall, check that day's menus, and generally make a pest of myself to the working staff. I was still relatively young for this facility, obnoxious, and opinionated. Overall, I was not fully appreciated for my general desire to be home and fully recovered. My family visited often. My daughters, my mom, and my long-suffering wife all kept me going throughout this time. My days were filled with great tedium and apathy concerning my slow progress and seeming inability to get better.

It takes time and constant effort to build strength that had been lost over 5 months of inactivity. I had spent far too much time laying in bed and watching daytime TV. I looked forward to the daily workouts in physical therapy where I worked to walk between two parallel bars or take a step up the stairs. Stairs were particularly difficult since I could only use my right leg to carry my weight. But I was getting better...

Essentially, my days were filled with getting up at 4:00 AM going up and down the hallways, having breakfast, and then watching TV until somebody came to visit, or physical therapy began. No Doctors visited, and the staff were knowledgeable but damn busy. Things progressed, with my gaining strength, when a catastrophe happened. Late on a Friday night, the trapeze above my bed collapsed and my bed split in half. I buzzed the night staff for help.

When they finally arrived, they looked confused and said their maintenance man had already left for his weekend. I realized that were going to do nothing to remediate the room. I can have a sharp and assertive nature, but I had been holding myself back from offering anything to the people who had a routine that they were obliged to follow, but this was beyond my patience.

I suggested, based on my experience as a facilities management professional that they call the man in on overtime to do the repairs. They stated that they were not allowed by the management to use overtime in any way. At this point, I finally lost my temper and suggested, using the most colorful language possible, that they needed to get the repairs done soon, or I would use my talents to sue the hell out of them and their facility. They called the owner and got them to agree to use overtime to get the repairs done.

Relatively soon, they suggested that I was well enough to go home. However, this was not their final attempt to get even. When I went to pay the final bill, they had charged me for that day and all the overtime that had occurred.

I, of course, refused to pay for both that day and all the overtime. They tried to make a fuss about the costs being mine to pay for all their effort. I handled it without a lawyer and just suggested that we were both better off to just ignore the day and costs involved. Within the month, they agreed to drop the matter.

My wife took me home...

It may seem like I survived my condition in good spirits, but it is far from the truth. I was depressed. My career was essentially over, and I was crippled with very debilitated muscles. I had always prided myself on the ability to overcome issues and look at the bright side of things.

My orthopedic surgeon even commented on how difficult it was for him to visit patients in the hospital. They were always hurt and depressed. He said it was a pleasure to see me because I was usually so upbeat and looking to do what I had to do to get better. By the time I was in Rehabilitation, that perspective had vanished. I was now obviously an invalid, and my persona had taken a massive blow, I now realized that my life had changed forever.

My wife was my anchor and was constantly supportive during this process. She knows me well enough to know when I am in a funk and covering up my depression. She helped with re-examining my life and told me that my life could easily start over. I had my brain, tremendous daughters, grandchildren, and herself.

My career was over, but there were many things I was still capable of doing. In other words, you're "alive and kicking", so quit being a baby and looking at things negatively. My wife, who knows exactly how to get me to fight and struggle to both survive and get better, used her verbal skills to goad me into improving. I needed to reinvigorate my approach fight for my life and return to the land of the living. I decided to write my first book, which is based on my experiences in the hospital during my hip problem. I have since written four books, counting this one in the total, and realized I "spin a yarn" if I put my mind to it.

I still had a lingering desire to return to the vision that I had had when I died on the operating table. I had been at one with the universe and floated in space among the planets and stars. I felt I could swirl the firmament with my hands, and I could still summon that vision, and I enjoyed that feeling very much.

It gave me a feeling that death was not an end, but an experience that we all would go through. Even though I did not fear this experience, I finally decided that this world was enough. I had things that still needed to be done, and my return to the cosmos could wait.

I also told an ICU nurse about part of my out-of-body experience, where I floated out of the hospital and hovered above the building. I mentioned that I saw a red sneaker at the edge of the roof. She looked startled when I told her about it, and she said, "Who told you about the red shoe?" I said I saw it when I was floating around. She gasped a little and never asked me again. I found out later that it is something they ask when someone claims to have an out-of-body experience. Evidently, I gave the right response before they even asked.

I restarted my life and desired to get better and better. However, when I returned to my residence, I found the house in total disarray. My wife had wanted me to stay in rehabilitation because she worried that if I fell, she would never be able to help me up. The house looked like a disaster. She was in the process of remodeling the downstairs to accept a hospital bed, but she had also decided that it would have to be completely repainted. There was no room for even my wheelchair to move around.

After moving things around and moving some things to the garage, we finally had one room set up for me to live. I was in seventh heaven to be home and in my own new hospital-type bed. I took some oxycodone and finally went to bed in my new hospital bed. My wife had purchased it second-hand, and I went to sleep in my own home for the first time in 6 months. I also had a brand-new lift chair that could help me stand up.

Now, I have begun the tough process required for full recovery. My wife was still working, so she needed to find someone who could keep me under control and out of trouble while she was teaching. Luckily, she found a local school bus driver who would sit in the house and help on occasion to keep me from falling over and would allow me to sleep in my massage chair until I would be able to move around unassisted.

I was also comforted by our dog, who normally avoided me at all times, but now insisted on sitting on my lap on the massage chair and just loved taking care of me by just being petted. She was a good dog and I felt especially close to her after I recovered because she wanted to help make me better. I still fell over several times, due to my insistence that I could do things before I really could. Once I hit my head on the stairs and probably rang my bell and passed out momentarily. I learned what I could no longer accomplish easily and reoriented my existence to my capabilities.

Now, I had been prediabetic before I became sick. Because my weight had increased to 280 pounds due to water retention and inactivity in the hospital, I became officially diabetic and could control it with either metformin or eventually glipizide. In the hospital, they could not be bothered with using glipizide, so I was put on insulin, after any meal.

I looked at it as just more times I was being poked and then injected with more drugs. I don't think it really helped me, but it was protocol. I prefer to control my blood sugar with exercise and minimal drug intervention, but exercise was no longer possible for me.

Since the operation, I have required minimal doses of insulin to maintain my health. Overall, my endocrinologist is very pleased with all my efforts in this regard. Also, I think it was a long-ago effect caused by my original career as a chemist and some of the more stupid decisions I made as a youth. I regret much of my early career when I used chemicals indiscriminately. Oh well, to be youthful and think yourself immortal is a tragedy for each generation, and not just my burden to bear.

THE REASONS
I AM THE WAY I AM

I was also comforted by our dog, who normally avoided me at all times, but now insisted on sitting on my lap on the massage chair and just loved taking care of me by just being petted. She was a good dog and I felt especially close to her after I recovered because she wanted to help make me better. I still fell over several times, due to my insistence that I could do things before I really could. Once I hit my head on the stairs and probably rang my bell and passed out momentarily. I learned what I could no longer accomplish easily and reoriented my existence to my capabilities.

Now, I had been prediabetic before I became sick. Because my weight had increased to 280 pounds due to water retention and inactivity in the hospital, I became officially diabetic and could control it with either metformin or eventually glipizide. In the hospital, they could not be bothered with using glipizide, so I was put on insulin, after any meal.

I looked on it as just more times I was being poked and then injected with more drugs. I don't think it really helped me, but it was protocol. I prefer to control my blood sugar with exercise and minimal drug intervention, but exercise was no longer possible for me.

Since the operation, I have required minimal doses of insulin to maintain my health. Overall, my endocrinologist is very pleased with all my efforts in this regard. Also, I think it was a long-ago effect caused by my original career as a chemist and some of the more stupid decisions I made as a youth. I regret much of my early career when I used chemicals indiscriminately. Oh well, to be youthful and think yourself immortal is a tragedy for each generation, and not just my burden to bear.

I was always fascinated by the sea and by chemistry. I grew up on a beach in Puget Sound and had always wanted to be involved with the sea. I graduated with a Bachelor of Science in chemical Oceanography, but when I was set to graduate, I went down to look at what jobs were available for Chemical Oceanographers, and they all seemed to be GS-4 (Talk about low pay) and required 6 months on a research ship at sea. I went to see a counselor, who determined that I had the credits for a degree in chemistry, but I needed to take freshmen English, a foreign language (German, French, Spanish, or Russian), and differential equations.

I had already taken three years of Spanish and could not hold a decent conversation, so I chose Russian. Big Mistake! The first day I learned that even the alphabet was against me. It had three types of symbols: Friends, Neutrals, and Enemies. The friends looked like our alphabet and sounded like them. The neutrals were entirely new symbols that I had to learn, and the enemies were those that looked the same but sounded entirely new. Thus, CCCP becomes SSSR in English. I suddenly saw why all Russian athletes wore CCCP on their sports jerseys. Also, Americans when trying to pronounce the Russian language sound like a chainsaw. I can still read some Russian, but I never got conversational. Real Russian native speakers sound truly amazing, almost musical with their expressions and use of language. I can see why many Russian poets exist and are very famous.

Then, I asked why I needed to take differential equations and I was told that I couldn't pass Physical chemistry without taking differential equations. When I pointed out that I had already passed Physical Chemistry, I was told that it would be "good for me". I realized that he was not going to give any waivers on the requirements, so I went on to say I would do it all.

As a senior, I went back and sat with freshmen in beginning English, I took Russian and took the required differential equations. I still wake up 45 years later with a nightmare about missing my differential equations final and failing the class. I somehow passed the class, though my heart was not in studying differential equations at all.

The upshot of all this information was when I started my job, toluene was not considered to be dangerous. Benzene was considered carcinogenic, but xylene and toluene were considered to be much more innocuous. Potentially damaging chemicals were not well understood at this time. In fact, I took an Organic Lab, where you had to identify the unknown chemical, you were given. One professor suggested that we taste it because they never give anything dangerous to undergrad students.

I was a definite individual in college who dramatically changed from being a bookworm and began to experiment with life in general and participated in many activities. I still managed to study enough to maintain an above-B average in all my courses which led to two Bachelor of Science degrees. One In Oceanography and my second in Chemistry. I graduated to my parent's relief after five years in college. My birthday was June 9th, my graduation was June 11th, and I started work on the 13th. So, you can see I was driven to succeed.

My first job out of college involved developing adhesives for the 'Do it Yourself'' market. I was immersed and involved with chemicals including vinyl acrylics and water-based acrylics. We rarely used gloves and I had it all over my hands and the only way to get it off was to wash them with toluene. I went from that exposure to working as a plant manager for a company that foamed the inside of a culvert pipe assembly with poly-isocyanate foam. Mono-isocyanates were considered to be carcinogenic, but the poly-isocyanates we used were just fine. (later found to be not true)

But I was a newly divorced single parent and desperately needed a job, any job. A pattern is emerging in my apparent "dumbness". I was not stupid, but I was committed to working to keep what remained of my family together. I am incredibly proud of both my daughters and what they have achieved with their lives.

This was far before I discovered the love of my current wonderful wife. She is the mother of my youngest daughter, and that daughter now lives about ten minutes away from my house. She and her husband are committed professionals, who have two of our many grandchildren. This makes us capable of being used as emergency babysitters on occasion.

The final personal issue was I was standing about 30 meters away from a huge pipe foaming operation when a small seam opened and ejected a stream of hot foam that hit me in the head. I panicked because the foam had coated my head, nostrils, ears, eyes and was expanding remorselessly. My only solution was to walk over to a drum of trichloroethylene stick my head in the open drum top and scrub the expanding foam from my head. I lost much of my hair after this occurred and I am convinced that this ultimately led to much of this story.

Just a little more background before we get back to the story. When my first wife left me, I was a single parent to my daughter. I needed to work as much as I could to keep my family alive. I decided to apply for a job at the local Navy base, but I ran into an innovative manager who always looked downstream for your overall capabilities. I was overqualified for the position but I began to work on the anti-corrosion efforts required at the base. Through an amazing series of events, I worked my way up from temporary painter, to supervisor, and then manager of a 175-person working group. As I moved up in the organization, I was increasingly called upon to help write proposals for working with the Navy. Eventually, I was spending 40 hours a week managing my group and 20-30 hours a week writing proposals. This became a crushing burden, and I am sure led to my self-destructive behavior, and infection, and ultimately led to the complete loss of my hip.

My trip back from the cruise where I developed my hip infection is still a blur to me. I was taken to LAX by a close friend of my wife, who lived in LA at the time. Luckily, she knew every backroad from the cruise terminal to the airport, otherwise, we would have missed our flight entirely. My wife threw me in a wheelchair, threw my bag on my lap, and ran to the TSA.

I went through TSA in a fog. We ran with the wheelchair to the gate, when my wife said, "Where's your bag?" My response was "What bag". So, she parked me at the gate and ran back to TSA to get my bag. Luckily, we had a friend who was a flight attendant, and he was on our flight. He helped me get out of the wheelchair and into the seat. He also helped me get off the plane and into the wheelchair to our car.

The trip from the airport to the hospital was another blur. All I could do was stare out the window and watch the highway signs pop when I saw them. Since I had received a morphine shot when I left the ship, I attribute that effect to the drug. I would see the sign, knew it was approaching, and then it would pop and get double in size. I can still remember the effect, which I thought was magical.

We got to the hospital, which is a huge one in Seattle. They had zero rooms available at the time, but they told me I was number 1 for the next room available. They told me that I was septic, and they could see my organs beginning to shut down. The danger did not make any sense to me, I was in a hospital; I should be able to survive. I looked over at my fellow patients in emergency. There was one fellow who was still bleeding from a knife fight in Pioneer Square. The nurse told me he was number 2. Knowing how first aid mandates the worst person always goes first, and he was still bleeding; I realized "I was in serious danger".

During this entire travel process, I could not have survived without my savior, my loving wife of 41 years. Without her help to get me to the hospital, I would not be alive. It is very important to me that I identify all the things that she did for me, to me, and that still does to keep me alive. Without her, I would not be here to write or continue to support my family in all their many efforts in life. She is the unsung hero of the story.

RETURN TO THE SCENE
AT THE TIME

Anyway, back to the main line of the story. I was scheduled for monthly blood tests to determine if I was infection-free. I could not receive an artificial hip until I could show the complete absence of infection in my hip. I used antibiotics, acupuncture, Chinese herbs, massage therapy, and holistic medicine. In other words, anything I could think of to turn my life around. I was unemployed, fighting enormous medical bills, handicapped, using painkillers, and still infected by staph.

So, I tried everything I could think of to remove the last vestiges of the infection. In the process, my doctors were checking my blood for continuing signs of infection. Then, they noticed that my liver readings were steadily showing signs of imminent failure. Both my albumin and bilirubin readings were increasing constantly. My liver doctor said he could see no long-term good prognosis for the liver. That due to my past exposure to chemicals and my diabetes, I was developing what he termed "Fatty Liver" and I would need a transplant within a few years. Not what I was looking for at all.

I also had one more challenge at this time. While I had been in the hospital with my hip, the company that I had been working with informed me by telephone that I had been fired and no longer had health insurance. Once I could use a walker for short distances, I took a double prescription of my painkillers and went to consult a lawyer. She developed a simple letter and sent it to the company, who agreed to pay back wages and allowed me to go on the Government COBRA program for health insurance. That is another long story, that I won't go into the details here.

A TRIP TO PARADISE

It took a very long time for me to get on the transplant list and my liver doctor (I had many doctors by this time) said I would have to have exceptional luck, since my state (Washington) is in the group with California, Oregon, Idaho, and Alaska).

Thus, there were many potential recipients, and my chances of finding a liver were not very good. I said to myself, do the best you can with what you've been given. See the doctor, follow all the instructions, and keep your hopes up. I had been retired on disability for several years after my hip replacement and we determined to use our savings to visit my wife's family in Hawaii. While I was there, I was involved with dynastic situations, caused by the soon-to-be eventual passing of my father and mother-in-law and their requests for how their legacy would be apportioned between the remaining four children.

My father-in-law was a revered Hawaiian elder, who still spoke Hawaiian and believed in Mana as well as Christianity. His surname was Kaanana, which is a shortening of the term Kahuna Anana, (in Hawaiian beliefs these were the priests that could pray you to death). He was always considerate to me, but I became obsessed with protecting my family from evil influences. Going to sleep at night, I would imagine that I was creating a force field around the earth to protect it from all evil influences and alien invaders. Crazy, but he had a very powerful personality, and I was just trying to survive.

We had to return to Hawaii several times to help the family, with my father-in-law eventually confined to a hospice facility due to cancer. In addition to my wife trying to help her parents cope with their situation, her father became debilitated by the massive metastasized cancer, and her mother became more demented, there was a power struggle over the house and inheritance. The elder sister wanted to continue to live in the house rent-free and had tried to have all of the property quit-claimed to her.

There was much love, deceit, and skullduggery going on internally within the family. I told my wife that it did not involve me, since it was her inheritance and not mine. We were ensconced in the small cabin in the backyard. I was still having a problem walking very far without assistance. But the sister made it plain that we were not to use the garage or certain parking areas because her husband needed to use them. This necessitated parking in subprime spots and walking to the back cabin. We were not allowed to use the main house for most things.

Her husband and my brother-in-law had retired as the chief of the Kauai Airport Fire Department and were fully qualified EMTs. I was still extremely vulnerable to high temperatures, and he was very helpful to me personally on those occasions. The rest of the time he was an SOB.

While my wife was helping her parents cope with the situation, I developed severe pain in my stomach, which was aggravated by constipation. My wife tried her best to relieve my pain, but we finally went to the urgent care facility, which scheduled an ultrasound and then a CAT scan of my belly. Although the technician told me that he was not allowed to tell me any diagnosis, he admitted to me that I had a gallstone that he saw with the scan.

I decided to follow my wife's advice, who had originally told me to go to the hospital. I asked the urgent care people to forward the images to the hospital. I then had her drive me to the emergency room. After waiting over two hours, I was finally introduced to a lady at the emergency room, who asked about my pain. She then had to check all my insurance to make sure that I could pay for anything that would be required. This took several hours. I was checked into the hospital, but no rooms were available, so I was parked in a hallway close to the emergency until a doctor saw me and finally got me into a room.

Even though I had grown to hate hospitals in general, the Hawaii hospital had a group of extraordinary nurses, who did their very best to make me comfortable. The doctor who had been assigned to me said they needed to perform an immediate operation to blast the stone with ultrasound and get it to pass. He also told me that the images showed not only a gallstone blocking the canal, but he thought that much of the pain was actually coming from the pancreatic duct, which is adjacent to the gall duct.

He also told me that the pain would subside after the gallstone was removed, but the gallbladder was full of additional stones that would eventually also cause future blockages, so did he have permission to schedule a second surgery to remove the entire gallbladder. He said they could do it simply with a series of holes that would allow them to encapsulate the gallbladder and then remove it easily.

Finally, I was sent to a room in the hospital. I was shocked to find myself alone since the hospital was supposed to be full to the brim. I had been scheduled to receive lithotripsy, the ultrasound destruction of the gallstone itself, which hopefully would allow relief from the pain. The operation would take place in the morning at 7:00 AM, so I would need to be up by 5:00 AM undergoing preparation. At 9:00 PM, a new patient was wheeled into the room, which I didn't mind at all since I knew the hospital was full. In fact, I had been expecting it since I arrived.

The nurses wheeled him to the bed by the window, since I was still in much pain, and didn't need a view. I tried desperately to try and return to a troubled sleep, due to the pain and knowledge that tomorrow I would be upon the operating table. My roommate decided he wanted to watch TV.

That was tough, but it was just as much his room as mine. But then he found an infomercial that covered all the songs from the 1960s and 1970s. They wanted you to buy the package of 10 songs for a low monthly fee. But they also insisted on playing portions of the songs they were selling. My roommate gradually increased the volume levels of the program and then proceeded to sing very loudly (in and out of tune) to every song that was being marketed.

After struggling for over ten minutes, I rapped on the dresser in between our curtained room, looked around the curtain, and asked politely if "he would mind turning down the volume since I had an operation early the next morning?" He responded with "Sure." The volume reduced and I went back to trying to fall asleep.

A minute later, I heard a commotion from the other side of the curtain. I heard the bed table thrown against the wall, followed by a loud exclamation that "No old man was going to tell me to turn it down." I knew I was in trouble and immediately pushed the button for the nurse.

When she arrived, the other patient continued to badmouth me, the hospital, and life in general. The nurse called for support and two more nurses arrived to try and calm the patient down. He continued to berate everyone, even pushing one of the nurses down.

The nurses decided that I was endangered but had no space available to put me. They parked me in the antechamber of a lady who did not want a male in her room at all. I was told to be very quiet and just wait. Eventually, the security people were brought in and one of them calmed him down.

He was a mental patient, who was not supposed to be left alone, with continuing observation. The charge nurse for that floor finally said she would stay with him in an isolation unit, as long as she had a pager that connected directly to security. Finally, at 2:30 in the morning, I was allowed to go back to my room. After about two hours of uninterrupted sleep, I was prepped for that morning's treatment.

After the treatment, the pain subsided quickly, and I was preparing for the good life in Hawaii once again. The surgeon arrived and said they wanted to perform laparoscopic surgery to remove the gallbladder itself because they had determined that it was packed with more stones and would just lead to another event of blockage in the near future. With no real options, I agreed to the surgery. I slept better than I had for a week since the pain in my stomach had subsided, and I thought I could live fine without a gallbladder, just change my diet a little bit.

Two days later, I was sedated and in the operating room. They installed three holes in my stomach and removed the gallbladder quickly and easily. I had three small bandages, and I could get around fine. I even went down and took a shower because the bandages were waterproof.

My favorite Hawaiian cousin delivered some handmade chocolates, which I immediately distributed to all the nursing staff who helped me during my stay. The candy was a big hit because I don't think anyone had ever given such a generous gift to them in the past. My cousin's chocolates were always a big hit because they were homemade and were made to look like real full-size credit cards. I was getting ready to check out of the hospital, after only a week. A new record for me. Then I had a last-minute visit from my surgeon who had removed the gallbladder. He gave me my last disturbing news. My liver was so damaged that every time he even touched the liver during the gallbladder removal, it bled and frequently had to be cauterized. He stated that if he had known how bad my liver already was, he would not have operated at all. His final advice was to get a transplant as soon as I could, or I would be dead very soon. He had a great bedside manner to tell me that I would be dead soon, but it was something I had to hear.

NEW HIP BLUES

Before the doctor arrived, I got to have the greatest pleasure of my life. The hospital had a walk-in shower, and the holes in my torso had been covered by waterproof tape. I went down and thoroughly washed my body and shampooed my hair.

For the first time in Hawaii, I felt clean and healthy. As I recalled earlier, he told me more about my condition. The doctor told me more why he told me to get on the transplant list, "The operation went well, but if I had seen how bad your liver was, I would never have operated this way. Every time I even brushed up against your liver, it bled, and we had to cauterize the bleeding. This required a lot of time. Your liver is beyond the 'fatty liver' and is fast approaching becoming cirrhotic."

I responded with, "What can I do?"

"You need a transplant as soon as you can," was all he said as he signed my discharge papers. In other words, "not my problem" - you take care of it.

Then he was out the door.

When I went home, I made an immediate appointment for a blood test and an appointment with my liver doctor. He looked at my results and pulled out all the stops and immediately put me on the liver transplant list. This meant a separate visit to the one major hospital in Seattle that does liver transplantation. I had to meet with a social worker, and their liver doctors and answer a thousand questions about my past. The main ones involved,

1. Were you an alcoholic?
2. Did you use drugs?
3. Have you met with others that need a transplant?
4. Have you taken the class that transplant patients are required to take?
5. What is your family's hereditary makeup?
6. Can you get to the hospital within three hours of the notification that an organ is available?

I signed up to take the course, where I met dozens of people who looked grey and close to death. There were several requirements for being on the transplant list:

You had to:

- Take the transplant class.
- Meet with a social worker once a year.
- See the transplant doctors regularly (usually every 3 months).
- Take a blood test every month.
- Stay within three hours of a transplant center at all times.
- Reduce my weight in any way I could.

I started to exercise daily. I could not walk, but I did have a recumbent bike that did not require me to stand and put any pressure on my still recalcitrant hip joint. I found that it was beyond me to return to anything like my previous activities. I had just enough energy for my regularly scheduled blood tests/doctor visits.

While I was in the hospital, the company that I had been working for fired me (illegally) and thus ended my insurance coverage. This was immensely stressful for my wife, who was being barraged by the hospital concerning my seemingly endless bills.

When I was terminated, I immediately started on COBRA insurance, but even though I made regular payments, their system would not declare me to have insurance when the hospital demanded payment. I finally called a retired friend who knew how the system worked and she got me straightened out. (Thank God.)

This also necessitated me locating an attorney to write a letter to my company and get them to rescind the termination. This got me the backpay involved but also soured me on continuing to work for them in any capacity. I was now probably going to be listed as permanently disabled.

My orthopedic surgeon was seeing me regularly to determine if I was eliminating the infection, but it seemed that I still had vestiges of the staph infection in my blood. He could not give me a prosthetic hip until I was infection-free. I tried all the antibiotics available to me and decided to try some Eastern medicine. I went to see a holistic Chinese medicine healer who thought he could help. I went to see him, and he held my wrist and forearms while he checked my chi. He had me stick out my tongue and then held up a mirror and showed me that it was dark black.

He suggested some very strong Chinese herbs, acupuncture, and massage therapy. I looked forward to my weekly massages and acupuncture treatments and took my Chinese herbs with a little lemonade mixture to kill the horrible taste. It took several months, but I began to get better and stronger. Then one day, I met with my liver doctor and got my latest results. No real improvement, but on the way home, I began to feel very weak.

The main problem was none of my insurance would cover the costs of Chinese medicine therapy. My Western doctors had virtually given up on ridding me of the infection, but that didn't matter to the insurance companies.

TRANSPLANT BLUES AND BEYOND

When I arrived in my driveway, I could not get out of the seat in the car. My phone was in the other seat, but I was too weak to even reach for it. I finally got the car door open and tried to stand up; I collapsed. Luckily for me, a neighbor was setting up his boat nearby and looked over at me collapsed next to my car. He called to his wife to help him get me up. They grabbed my arms but couldn't lever me up. I had them call an ambulance and they arrived in less than ten minutes.

I was delirious by this time, so they took me directly to the hospital. I remember that trip as if I was in a fog. In other words, not very well. I remember the ambulance people asking me a lot of questions, and I don't think I handled the questions very well.

When I got to the hospital, I was wheeled into a room where they asked me many questions.

Who is the President? My answer was "I think it's Bill Clinton" (it was Barack Obama at that time). I had celebrated Obama's election and was committed to change in America.

What year is it? I think it is 1995 (it was probably 2012).

Various other questions that I gave truly nonsensical answers to..., but I did tell them that I had been having pain in my tooth. They took an x-ray, and it showed an abscess.

Although I was delirious, I did see them look furtively at each other and kind of roll their eyes. They did a quick blood culture and found a high count of white blood cells. They decided that I was septic again, so they tried an immediate antibiotic for strep, hoping that the tooth had abscessed and that it was strep this time and not staph, which would have been much more dangerous.

After one day of intravenous antibiotics (specifically for strep), I responded and answered all their questions correctly. They gave me a prescription for an oral antibiotic and let me go to a dentist to deal with the tooth. Within the week, I had the tooth pulled and within two weeks, I was off the antibiotics and back to full recovery.

It was relatively scary to be back in the hospital, but I was very glad that they and I responded so quickly, and within a few days, I was home again. I continued bi-weekly acupuncture and Chinese herbal treatments. I could drive a car but was not fully capable of doing that in a reasonable fashion. I was stopped by a Sheriff when I was a mile from my house. I was given a sobriety test, which I passed, but he said I should be more careful and just go home. I was taking oxycodone on a regular basis (about every 4-6 hours). I needed it throughout the day because I was still in pain from my hip surgery.

I especially needed it to sleep at night. I noticed that I was needing it more often and that it was not as effective as it had been. I looked up the information and found that it was a strong narcotic, even though I was told it was not an opioid. Also, I was followed by an old friend's children in their car; and my friend called to tell me that I had been driving very erratically. He was very concerned about my health.

After throwing up in my mom's house and in her car, I decided to stop taking the oxycodone entirely. I would go "cold turkey". Within two days, I was beginning to suffer withdrawal. I couldn't sleep at night, and spent 5 days watching late-night TV, shivering in my massage chair, and being a cast-iron SOB to my wife. She worried about me, but she knew I needed to break the habit and was very thoughtful and encouraging, as she saw me struggle through this episode of withdrawal.

I began to itch all over and could not concentrate at all. I could read and couldn't even watch TV. I just sat in my massage chair and sweat. Even the dog, who had always tried to comfort me when I was ill, stayed away from me during this withdrawal. Finally, I overcame my need for the drug; and I gave my excess pills to an old friend, who used them to get her roof completely repaired. I found I didn't care if she didn't use them herself.

My life settled into a routine of doctor visits, learning to walk, building strength in my now flaccid muscles on my recumbent bike, and watching daytime TV. My wife was not retired and was still working daily teaching music in a local public school. That was one attractive part of my life at this time; I had been declared permanently disabled from the hip repair and was now on Social Security and Medicare. I added a supplemental plan to get better benefits.

Within the next year, I obtained new blood tests every month that tracked my liver enzymes. My liver doctor informed me that I had six months to a year before the liver would fail and his only long-term hope for me was to get a transplant. He was not very encouraging in that prospect, since he stated that my state was in the same group as Oregon, Idaho, Alaska, and California. So, my chances of competing for a viable liver were not that great. Since I still seemed to be healthy at that time, I started consulting family members for possibilities.

Even though partial transplants of livers can be quite successful, the University of Washington Medical Center suggested that I needed a complete liver transplant. Suddenly, they called that I had hit the lottery, and a new liver was available. The identified liver came from a former drug addict and an alcoholic. Because it was from a compromised liver, I refused the offer and potentially signed my own death warrant.

Then, beyond reason, they found another liver. I thought, "How lucky can I get?" Unfortunately, when they called me, I had contracted a raging case of the flu. They refused to consider me capable of receiving the liver, so I went back on the transplant list. I was terribly disappointed but also relieved. A liver transplant is a horrendous operation with a steep recovery curve.

THE HEROINE
OF THE STORY

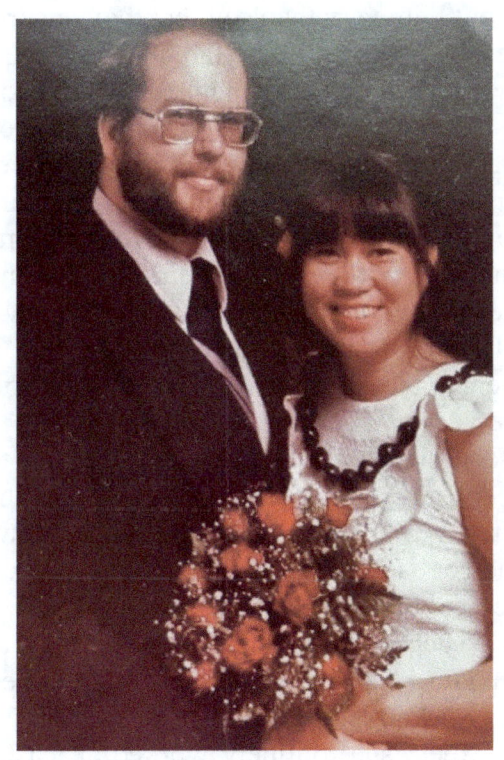

Our Wedding Photo

I need to express my wonder that, luckily, I fell in love with someone who not only took care of me but was instrumental in my survival.

We met over forty years ago when I asked her to dance and then the band took their break. Instead of walking away, I sat down. I'm sure she thought that it was assertive of me to ask her to dance and then sit down, but that was me at that time. Eventually, we danced the night away and I asked her to meet me the following night for dinner. She was careful to accept cautiously and make sure that we met in a neutral location so she could escape if she needed to.

We had a nice time. Evidently, I intrigued her enough that we began to go out regularly. She was a Hawaiian/Chinese American from Hawaii. She was born in Honolulu, and I was a somewhat misplaced Alaskan who had been born in Fairbanks. The strains of fate that allowed us to meet in a rural town in Washington are mystical to me, but I am very thankful that they occurred when they did. I was a recently separated single father and working at a job that I didn't like. I was also soon to be unemployed, due to a layoff.

Nevertheless, I soon proposed to her, and she accepted. I had to explain that I was not totally free yet, since my divorce had not been finalized at that time. She understood, and we went through the divorce from my previous wife together. We got married when the divorce was finalized, and my three-year-old was included in the ceremony. She even got her own ring in the ceremony. My wife had already made plans for a summer vacation in Europe, and I still had a new job to prepare to accomplish and needed to continue to take care of my three-year-old at home.

She was a schoolteacher who used the summer to expand her horizons, and I encouraged her to keep at it. I don't think she cared if I approved or not. She loves to travel and see new cultures and sights. When she got back, we began our life together. She and I had another daughter, about four years after we married.

I was driven to succeed in my job as a manager for a maintenance company working on a Navy Submarine Base. I worked 60-70 hours a week. While as a schoolteacher she was not required to work more than 40 hours a week, she routinely worked at least 50 hours per week (as most teachers do).

After putting up with my work schedule for many years and watching my mood increase whenever I was stressed, she demanded we take a three-day cruise vacation to Mexico. With my usual bad grace about taking time off, I went on the cruise. I fell ill on the cruise, and she used all her skills to get me through the cruise, not only taking care of me on the ship, but she got me back to a major hospital in Seattle, where I was diagnosed with Septicemia.

For the next five months, she saw me through three major operations, death, ICU, weird hallucinations, drug addiction, and eventually even more hospitalizations. She slept in the hospital, sometimes on the ledge of my room. She continued to work at her job, handling my care and the insurance situations that were nearly insurmountable.

The company I was working for at that time fired me (illegally); so, I lost my insurance. This required my wife to undergo additional stress since the hospital wanted either insurance or major payments constantly. All the time staying as upbeat as she could with events that would have crushed many people. I spent many hours just lying in a hospital bed, hoping that I would get better someday. My career had ended, and I was crippled, and out of work. Not exactly the life I had promised her when we got married.

I don't want to give the impression that my wife is a saint. She definitely is not. Cross her and find out. She is known in my family for going "Nuclear" if she is stymied. There is no easy way to negotiate with her. It's her way or she will declare war and take no prisoners. This can be tough to deal with at times, since there may not be a simple win-win solution in her skillset. In fact, she can be a cast iron SOB when she wants to be that way. That doesn't mean I don't love her more than I thought I could love, but it explains how she can achieve what she does.

There were many times in my rehab honestly where I just wanted to give up, but she wouldn't let me. She had already made the decision that I was "a Keeper", so she worked her hardest to get me well enough to continue. I owe her my life, so when she says we are going to enjoy the remaining years of our life together... I just say, "Yes Dear". She took over many of my previous functions around the house. She mows the lawn, does major repairs, pays bills, etc. She is amazing and deserves everything I can give her now and in the future. She is a delight, and I appreciate her strong will and effectiveness.

AIR AMBULANCE
ISSUES

Several times after I returned home, I fell. I am generally a klutz, but I have also lost some sense of balance after all the operations and illnesses. My worst fall took place in the downstairs living area of my home. I fell and hit my head and started bleeding all over the carpet. We called for the local ambulance, who picked me up for the 30-mile trip to the local emergency room. They checked my blood pressure while working to control the bleeding.

My blood pressure was extremely low, but my heart rate was elevated. The local hospital took a blood sample and realized that my liver was way out of whack. The hospital controlled the bleeding but then decided I needed much more serious attention than they could give. They called in an air ambulance to take me to the Seattle trauma center (Harborview Hospital).

The trauma center is usually working on patients that are "in extremis". I was not bleeding anymore, just incredibly "loopy". They took my history, did some quick bloodwork, and made a rational decision to send me off to the transplant unit and their associated hospital at the University of Washington Medical Center.

They already had me in their database as a needy liver transplant patient. They stabilized my chemistry with some very specific drugs, kept me a day, and then sent me home to await the more permanent solution of a liver transplant.

I was fine and happy to get home until I got the bill. "Wowza", I was impressed with what they thought of the price for helicopter services to avoid a ferry. This was something I really couldn't afford more than once. I have since purchased a MASA plan for emergency transport, whenever it might be required.

However, less than a year later, I was back in the hospital in Bremerton and was no longer responding to the prescriptions that saved me last time. The liver had obviously gotten much worse, and I was nearing my death from liver failure. The Bremerton hospital contacted the UWMC Transplant Department, who told them to ship me over right away. They might have a donor with a possible liver for me.

I flew out that hour, and that is a trip that I have absolutely no memory of; I think I was beyond caring about pretty much anything and very near death. My next recollection was a whole gaggle of doctors standing around my hospital bed and discussing what to do. I am sure there was a surgeon in charge, a transplant doctor, and a whole bunch of students.

The surgeon was a very competent lady surgeon, who asked if I would take any liver that would be offered. I found out later that my wife had already accepted those conditions, and this was mainly a formality for the paperwork. I knew I was close to death and had no choice except to proceed. I just said, "Sure, go ahead."

I was also nearly out of options since I was now really reacting to the abnormal functions of my diseased liver. My youngest daughter, who was in college in Olympia, came to see me. I think my wife told her that I was close to death. She arrived expecting to see the man who had taken her to gymnastics for seven years, supported her in all of her endeavors, and was always a rock of sane advice. What she saw instead was a bloated mass of protoplasm lying almost comatose in a hospital bed. When she came, I awoke and handed her a hospital brochure, saying, "Here's your mail." She held it together in the room, but later went out into the hallway and cried. She hadn't expected me to decline so rapidly. Also, I think my mom called my brother in Oregon to tell him that I didn't look very good and that it was time to come see me before the end.

He came up to visit, which I really appreciated. He sat in my hospital room and attempted to strike up a conversation, but I was really not capable of holding up my end of any conversation. He then tried to start a game of cribbage with me, but I found to my complete dismay that I couldn't even count my cards in the game, let alone use my pegs to advance on the board. Not a very pleasing experience for either of us.

It also showed my family that I was relatively crazy. There was even a point where I got up late one night and demanded that I go downstairs and use my massage chair. The nurse tried to calm me and told me that there were people in the room downstairs and I needed to return to my bed. I felt they were trying to control me and initially demanded that I be allowed to go downstairs.

I even tried to force my way by them. I was so incredibly weak by this time; I never would have succeeded. They finally got through to me and I returned reluctantly to my bed. I dreamed that night that there was a conspiracy to keep me in the hospital, drugged and they were tapping me to use my blood to develop some special drugs for people.

My wife watched me slowly decline further into delirium, without hope that I could recover. At the last minute, a liver was found. It was not from an alcoholic or drug addict, but it was from a deceased prisoner. The doctors informed me that I could accept or refuse. In my delirious state, my wife accepted it for me. They did ask me just before I went into the operation if I agreed. I remember saying "You bet'cha" otherwise I'm dead.

After an 8-hour operation, I awoke with a massive cut that looked like the "Mercedes" icon on my torso. Staples were everywhere along the cut and relatively no pain. But that was the first day of the recovery, the pain would arrive the next day.

The pain arrived in a massive way the very next day. I was still relatively insane, so it made it doubly harder to communicate what I needed to maintain any composure. Plus, they began administering the anti-rejection drugs immediately. I longed for any ability to get comfortable in a hospital bed, whose controls always seemed to be positioned in a way that I could not reach them or adjust them for any comfort.

After the operation, I was lying in bed recovering from the operation and examining the huge number of staples that covered my torso. Liver replacement involves what is called the "Mercedes cut" because the design it leaves resembles the logo for a Mercedes auto. I had been cut from my sternum to my belly button. Staples held the rolled-up skin layers together.

Every time I attempted to adjust my position in the bed, I would feel some part of the incision pull and feel the pain. After several days of using painkillers, I attempted to wean myself off them. I had encouragement from both my wife and my mom, but I was incapable of eliminating them from my recovery process. I needed them simply because the incision was so massive that I was incapable of dealing with the pain without them.

Plus, after a brief nap, I usually found staples had popped loose from the incision. This necessitated their reinstallation. Especially at the beginning of the recovery. Later in the process, it became routine to find several staples in my bed, but they no longer needed to be reinstalled.

I was given a button that would allow a modest dosage of painkillers to be administered intravenously. I found myself watching the clock for when the button would work again since it was limited to allow only a small amount of painkiller to be administered at any one time. Finally, they took the button away to ensure that I would have to request it each time. Thankfully, within 5 days, I no longer needed any painkillers.

A new issue arose in that I could not go to the bathroom, or even attempt to rise for the installation of a bedpan. Initially, this was not much of a problem since I was not eating and had a catheter for draining urine. But if and when I had to poop, I needed several people to help support me to get into a position to properly use a bedpan. I had no muscle control at all to help lift me onto a bedpan. I also tried several times to contact the nursing staff for help, but they did not respond quickly enough to avoid the issues created when they were late.

Many times, I could not hold it and made a mess out of my bed. I was in so much pain, I really didn't care about the mess. But it did mean a lot of extra work for the hospital staff.

They would have to roll my enormous carcass on its side, remove the sheet under me, and then roll me in the other direction to remove the sheet. The same process was used to install a new sheet. It certainly informed visitors how ill I was. I was not able to help myself. I went through this humiliating process for over three weeks, before I had healed enough to control some of my bodily functions, and it became easier to help the nursing staff with my care.

When I had recovered enough to try and use a bedside commode, a new issue occurred. As soon as I attempted to transfer to the chair, I went into uncontrollable seizures. My legs would start to shake and my arms would go spastic. Soon I was not even allowed to try and get out of bed without staged support by a cadre of nurses and orderlies.

One of the impacts of not being able to walk is that your body needs to get vertical and walk. It is definitely essential in the healing process. Not being able to walk also neutralized any hospital solutions for my care. I went into a type of suspended animation, where I didn't get worse, but I also did not improve. My sutures healed but I ballooned to over 280 pounds. A lot of the weight gain was just water because it hurt so much to try and go to the bathroom.

This alone was tough because I was mainly subsisting on mashed potatoes and Jell-O. All the other hospital food was completely unappetizing.

Just a little about hospital food:

a) It is usually bland and completely lacking in any seasoning.

b) It is almost always cold when it arrives after a long trip from the central kitchen to the orderlies who deliver it. I think that the kitchen staff at most hospitals do a wonderful job, but feeding thousands of patients on multiple floors and with conditions that are challenging, to say the least. It is darn near impossible to get food to individual patients in a fashion where it is hot and still somewhat appetizing. Understanding the difficulty involved does not make it easier to eat bland, tasteless, and cold food.

c) It also arrives usually when it's most inconvenient to eat. Either because you are scheduled to talk with doctors or have some MRIs, CAT scans, or an ultrasound to accomplish.

d) I found that I can subsist on mashed potatoes and gravy, and sugar-free Jell-O for a long time. This also makes dining on a cruise ship much more pleasurable in comparison. The food arrives hot and cooked to perfection and is exactly what you wanted.

I just grew to hate hospital food and have had a visceral reaction ever since. My sympathies to anyone who endured a long hospital stay and the need to eat hospital food for any length of time.

What ensued now was a long-term care situation in the hospital. Each new week allowed them to change the type and quantity of various medications, trying to find a combination that would allow my new liver to function without rejection, and that would allow me to walk without falling on my ass. Nothing seemed to work. I would spend the week trying the new combination of drugs. I would feel really good, and then they would gather six nurses and orderlies to help me up. Almost as soon as I tried to stand next to the bed, my legs would start to shiver and then spasm semi-rhythmically until I collapsed into their waiting arms. After the first 6 or 7 times, I no longer looked forward to trying to walk at all. So now I fell into what seemed to be an endless routine. I would wake up in the morning and wait until the kitchen would accept my orders, order scrambled eggs, sausage, then orange juice.

The phlebotomist would stop by to get their three vials of blood for the day's tests. I would see the morning round of nurses, where they would write down who was the RN and who was the LPN working that day's shift. They would also let me know who was scheduled for the night shifts. They would ask me what my goals were for that day. I got to be fairly callused after several weeks because it never changed. My goals did not change. I wanted to get the "heck" out of there. (actually, my language was far less decorous and very blunt). They eventually gave up and put my actual terms up on the wall.

Around 10, the doctor would come by on their daily rounds and listen to me complain for a while. It was a teaching hospital, so they usually had the doctor, several interns, and medical students in attendance around my bed. I was considered to be an "interesting" case and must have been a general enigma to most of the students.

First, because I was a successful transplant survivor of a liver transplant, not very common; but I also had a unique reaction to the anti-rejection drugs. The doctor would go to great lengths to properly instruct the various students in my personal eccentricities. I had learned much of the hospital terminology by now, so I could usually follow along with the conversation. The students asked many questions about the pharmacological complications, which I thought were very astute.

I began to long for the freedom to just get out of bed and walk to the bathroom. You never know what you will miss until it is taken away from you. I tried to treat each new drug regimen with hopeful optimism. As each new one was tested, I rose confidently out of bed, sure that this combination was going to work.

After each new test, where my legs would go into spasm and my arms would quiver like jelly, I would sink back onto my hospital bed and become very despondent. The doctors would come in and cluck their tongues in skepticism and go back to talk to their comrades and the pharmacists to look for some new approach. I was gradually losing hope that I was ever going to get better

SURVIVAL AND A NEW SURPRISE

So, to recap the previous chapter, whenever they tried to have me stand up to use my legs, I immediately went into seizures. My legs would violently tremble and spasm, to the point that I would collapse back onto the bed or onto the floor. Sometimes, all they had to do was suggest that I try to sit on the edge of the bed and the shaking and tremors would start. They decided that it had to be a reaction to the anti-rejection medicine. They and I were stuck in a hard place. I needed the anti-rejection medicines to keep my new liver, but the prescriptions being given caused a reaction that would not allow me to get better.

Now, there ensued a regular existence of a long time waiting for the incision to heal while I stayed horizontal. The human being is not designed to be horizontal for extensive periods of time. I was never comfortable with a line of over forty staples that covered me from the sternum to the belly button and across the line under my ribs. I couldn't move easily without feeling the staples pull at my skin. I was not allowed to move nor could I realistically. I had a catheter that was obtrusive, and which drained into a bag under the bed. I would not be allowed to leave until I could walk and defecate on my own.

At the cruise table, there were gasps as I told of both the transplant and the aftermath of seizures. They were amazed that I was able to get a transplant and that I was telling about both my luck and the absolute devastation that followed. That, along with still being alive to tell the story. Their lives and disappointments paled in comparison. They were triply shocked when I told them I was only a third of the way through my story. I began to continue the story, concerning the hospital's continuing efforts to solve my issues and get me up and running to my future.

What followed was five months of tedium, punctuated with bouts of disturbance. I was too sick and incapable of walking, so I was catheterized, which was not only painful but made urination extremely painful when it occurred. I complained bitterly to any nurse when they had time. I was just considered to be a complainer. Finally, a nurse checked on the installation and found that it had been installed backward. I have no idea what that means, so I didn't know that it could have been installed improperly. I just thought it was a drain, but once it was fixed, I became a much more complacent patient.

Now I was exposed to seemingly endless weeks of trial-and-error pharmacy, as the doctors tried to find some combination of anti-rejection medication that would work and still allow me to stand up and walk. Each week, I would try a new combination of drugs and they would watch me fall. They would shake their heads and talk to the pharmacist about what to try next.

What it meant to me was another week in the hospital to take new drugs and then try again. They would not remove the catheter until I proved I could walk to the bathroom. My family found it increasingly difficult to visit. It required preparation since it required car ferry traffic which is both expensive and difficult to plan. I still cherished each visit, since it broke up the tedium of daytime TV.

My mom would bring freshly cut-up watermelon pieces, sometimes daily. These I gobbled up with great pleasure compared to hospital food. I really treasured these visits and the break from the hospital food available.

I still had trouble sleeping in a hospital bed, though it greatly improved when my wife brought a pillow from home. Hospital pillows are the worst, because they don't scrunch, are flat, and never the right height to rest comfortably. Bed controls are consistently difficult to reach and control. Plus, I was on a watch list where every two hours they did a blood pressure and heart check. Every four hours I would have a blood glucose check. Thus, when I finally managed to get to sleep, I would be awakened and checked and then try to go back to sleep.

I tried using "Ambien" as a sleeping prescription. They found out I was extremely allergic to this drug. The one night I was given it, I hallucinated, grew violent, and had to be restrained. My wife had seen me delirious, sick, and in pain, but this scared her and made her wonder if I would ever be allowed to leave the hospital.

Daytime TV is exceedingly boring at best, but it was all I had. My family and friends tried their best, but they couldn't be there all day every day. I began to live for their visits and even the daily doctor visits and shift changes which brought in new nurses to entertain. When visits were expected and they couldn't make it, I became surly and depressed. After all, I had nothing else to look forward to and when they did not occur, I was upset. I wanted my wife to be there as much as she could, and she dreamed of a life that was not tied to a hospital. She had to work, maintain our house, take care of the dog, and try to get some time away from someone who was so needy.

I almost gave up. It was just so hard to recover all over again. The hospital had a chart on the wall that identified the nurses involved in my care for that day. It would identify who was RN and who was the LPN on duty. It also listed any events for that day. There was a space on the board for my own personal goals. As I stated earlier, I instructed them to always say that my goal, was to "Get the f#@$ out of here." This was most humorous to the staff and visitors. It also epitomized my overall attitude of being in the hospital for an indeterminate amount of time.

As much as I wanted to get out, it was apparent to everyone that I was not well enough to leave. My seizures occurred as soon as I tried to stand up. They changed the level of prescriptions every week, with no measurable improvement. My despair about being confined to a bed, without any ability to walk or change my position without help was devastating to me. I relished visits, whenever I had a visitor and treasured the times when my own family came daily to visit me.

So, now came the time of my most desperate feelings. It seemed that no matter how I approached my condition, there was no improvement. I almost lost hope that I would ever be allowed to leave the hospital. The bills kept piling up. They would change my type/quantity of medicines and then watch for my reactions as I tried my best to walk without collapsing. It never seemed to get any better. I gave up trying to improve and just waited for something to work. There seemed to be nothing that I could do.

I lashed out at family and friends. An old friend from college stopped by to see how I was. I could barely wave at him as he peeked around the curtain. He was an esteemed doctor in the UW health system. He was renowned for his knowledge of rehabilitation medicine and is the department head at Harborview Medical Center, but I couldn't even see him. My mom warned me about the dangers of painkilling medicine. I took affront at her reproaches and threw a protein bar at her.

I became inconsiderate of the time my wife and family needed to pursue their own priorities. Any delay, like a late ferry, or their own personal needs led me to blame them for any delay in their visits. I tried hard to understand that they couldn't be there if I was bored or depressed. I could be a complete ass to them on occasion. I created this book to apologize for any hard feelings that still exist.

After four months of not responding to the various combinations of drugs, they called in a young pharmacist who stated to me "Many times the new liver will take over all of the immune functions." He suggested that they reduce the anti-rejection drugs to almost nothing. The doctors, "being a conservative lot," would not go for a complete recession of all anti-rejection drugs. But they agreed to reduce it to the absolute minimum that protocol would allow. Within a week, I could walk feebly to the bathroom under close supervision.

Now that I could finally walk, I was subjected to the gentle ministrations of the physical therapists. They did their very best to help me regain some strength. They would arrive usually at the same time as my lunch and announce that they needed to get me to walk down the hallways. They would always check the oxygen percentage in my finger, make sure that I was 95% or better, and then get me in a cardiac walker to get some exercise.

They were reliably intense and serious about pushing me to do more. I resented it at the time since my food was invariably even colder when I returned, but it was exactly what was necessary for me to get any better. Although I hated them and physical therapy at the time, they were the best thing for me.

Within two weeks, I could walk down the hall and back. Many times, they would stay with me throughout the walks and then suggest that I attempt to sit in a chair instead of returning to the bed. They would then leave me sitting in the chair, out of reach of my buttons to summon help. Sometimes I would sit there for several hours before someone would check on me. By then I was exhausted and weak. Still, within three weeks, I could climb the makeshift stairs (four steps), without requiring a rest in-between.

My wife was concerned that I not be allowed to come home if I couldn't fend for myself. She still had to work, since she could not retire before she reached 62 and ½ years old. Finally, I got the approval of the physical therapists that it would be safe for me to go home. That I was as stable as they could make me. They couldn't justify to the hospital that I be retained further.

NEW TROUBLES TO SURMOUNT

Now the next wrinkles arrived. I was constantly being imaged by MRIs, CAT scans, or ultrasounds. They found residual evidence that at some point in the past, I had suffered a "minor ischemic event" (a stroke) so a new drug was administered called a statin as a preventative measure to ensure that I would not have another stroke. Also, they had been worried about the state of the new liver. They could not check it before it was transplanted, but it "might" contain a virus known to destroy kidneys. They had been watching my creatine levels rise for the past months, but now suspected that the damage was increasing, and it was probably caused by this virus.

By now the group at the table was aghast at what had been happening to me. Many of them could not believe that I had been subject to seizures and that it would take so many months to resolve. My wife spoke up then and said not only did it happen that way, but she almost lost hope that I was going to survive to come home. She stated, I saw him fall and not be able to control his legs at all. It was scary to see and not be able to help.

It also led to many occasions when I could not control my bowels, which made the nurses very unhappy because they had to deal with an overweight patient who was not very helpful. It would just happen, even if I had friends visiting. I could not control it at all. The nursing staff were already overworked and stressed and did not need the extra needs of a patient who could not control themselves.

I apologized repeatedly, but they couldn't understand why I couldn't control it. The doctor finally explained to them, concerning the anti-rejection drugs, that they were the problem. They became much more tolerant and understanding that I couldn't always control my body. The doctors thought I would get better as they adjusted the medicines, but it would take weeks or months. They resigned to help as much as they could, but they also had a floor of people who had their own issues.

One of my oldest and dearest friends came to visit me, and I had one of the episodes involving a complete collapse. I had been an upperclassman, and we had many fun times involving escapades in the dorms. To see me no longer being the image of calm but now almost incapable of living was a shock to her.

I now have a new kidney doctor assigned to my case. He was a pleasant young doctor, who said he got into nephrology because it usually did not require much after-hours work. He looked at my case history and thought I should get monthly checkups to watch for increasing kidney failure statistics. They never did improve, but I kept taking the medicine and hoping for some miracle.

ADDICTION
IS REALLY UGLY

While I was in the hospital, they began to use morphine to help control the pain in my hip. They felt that it would lead to long-term problems with addiction, so they switched me a supposedly superior and less addictive pain killer, oxycontin. This was not supposed to be an opiate, so would not cause any addictive problems for me. At least, that was what I was told.

Since I was taking oxycontin for pain, and to allow me to sleep through the painful nights, I didn't worry about its' long-term impact. Nor did I conduct my usual research on any chemical that I took. I just assumed that they were giving me a miracle drug that was really effective at reducing my pain and was allowing me to rest.

My wife and Mom all suggested that this was not really helping me, and they worried about its long-term effects. (This was long before it was understood that it was highly addictive. Doctors prescribed it for me for pain for over 11 months.) I noticed that I had several episodes of the onset of serious nausea and vomiting. After being on it for over 11 months, I realized that I had become quite dependent upon it for anything that I needed to accomplish. I even took a larger dose to be able meet with the lawyer who sent a letter to the company that had fired me for being sick. (I got a settlement of back wages)

I decided to quit taking the oxycontin entirely one night and within a day started suffering "the shakes" and insomnia for about a week. My wife was sure that I was going crazy. I was constantly shivering and could not get comfortable anywhere. But I avoided taking any oxycontin for the next week. My wife watched with concern while I shook and shivered for the next week; unable to sleep so I watched DVD after DVD, while sitting in my massage chair. I refused to give in to my insatiable desire to just take one more pill, because I needed to shake the drug off.

I did not see snakes or insects climb the walls, but it was very unpleasant during the process. I could not get comfortable no matter what my position or what was on TV. I watched TV without sleep for the entire week. I was in a fog for much of the time, and thankfully my wife watched over me and just encouraged my efforts to become drug free.

Finally, after a week, I was free of the drug's grip on my soul. After becoming free of the need for oxycontin, I ended up giving the remainder of my prescription to an old friend. She got her roof repaired by using them to get a work crew for free. That tells you both the street value of the drug and the current state of the construction industry.

Later, I spoke to my regular GP during my physical, who was astonished that I had quit cold turkey and said that they had some medicine that may have made it easier to quit. I thanked him for the offer, but I was over it by then and needed no further assistance. One thing that showed up during my physical showed that my liver was becoming a problem. He sent me to a liver specialist, who suggested that I would be needing a new liver in the near future (1-5 years).

HOME AT LAST AND HAPPY

I was finally allowed to go home. However, I still was required to go to the UW transplant center every month to be examined by my doctors. After five months, I got a letter from the doctors to allow me to jump the line at the ferry to get on the ferry without the long lines and significant waits involved. These documents can be difficult to obtain, but it went like clockwork and greatly eased my wife's life in overcoming my illnesses'.

What followed was relatively easy, I spent hours at home relaxing in my massage chair. Exercising to build strength. My wife had purchased a lift chair to allow me to stand without much effort and a hospital bed. She slept in the next room, so if I awoke, she could help with any needs.

What followed now was very tedious and mundane. I would arise in the morning after my wife had left for work. I would watch a little TV, followed by thirty minutes of exercise on my recumbent bike.

Around ten o'clock, the lady we hired would arrive to ensure that I did not fall during the day. She would fall asleep in a chair, while I made sure I did not fall in the downstairs living room. Later, after my caretaker had gone home to do her daily job, bus driving schoolchildren. I would complete another thirty minutes of exercise and then take a 1–2-hour nap and wait for my wife to come home and tell me about her day teaching music at an elementary school. This went on for several months. I began to get strong enough to drive short distances.

I recovered enough that I could drive the back roads to get to my blood tests. When it was required that I meet my doctors, my wife would take the day off and drive into the city. She would take me across the ferry, and do some shopping while I went through the necessary blood tests and medical appointments. She was always there with me to listen to the doctor's discussion of my future prognosis. My local liver doctor and the assigned transplant doctor were both pleased with my progress and the various measures of liver functions.

My new liver performed like a champ. My liver functions since the operation have all been exactly what my doctors expected. My body functions with the new liver and I have had no problems with any of my body chemistry for over 7 years. Well beyond the expected life of most transplant patients. I have had zero complaints about my liver. I never drank very much and now do not have alcohol or use any drugs beyond those taken to maintain the quality of the transplant. I take Tacrolimus, Tamsulosin, Calcium, Magnesium, vitamins, prednisone, and a statin for heart health. I also take a very expensive drug to help reduce potassium in my blood, which one of the previous medicines produces. My blood pressure is 115/77 and continue to work out at least an hour/day. I take every COVID vaccine/booster available. I am vaccinated against shingles, pneumonia, RSV, and flu. 'I continue to travel as much as I can and babysit my grandchildren on occasion.

DIALYSIS IS NEVER FUN?

However, the nephrologist was increasingly concerned with my creatinine readings. They were rising steadily and were gradually getting to the point where something would need to be done. He suggested either a kidney transplant or dialysis would be required soon. I was still producing urine, but the kidneys were no longer removing the byproducts that they normally would.

He thought a transplant was a long shot since I was already a liver transplant recipient, and I would need treatment before a kidney could be located. He found a dialysis chair available but it was over 60 miles from my house. All the other closer facilities were completely full, 24 hours a day. I asked when I would need to get started. He said immediately.

So, my wife would load me in her car every other day and drive the 60 miles to the facility, work out, and then pick me up to return 60 miles to our home. Not much fun, but I enjoyed my time with her in the car. Within weeks, I began to see why many dialysis patients finally just gave up and died. It seems endless, and you never escape long enough to feel normal. You are always undergoing dialysis, spending the next day recovering from dialysis and then you start all over again.

At this point, the audience at my cruise table groaned. Several commented that they had friends that went through dialysis and how unpleasant and ultimately unhelpful. After a few years of Dialysis, many just gave up. It was too difficult to go to dialysis every other day hoping you find a solution. Many just gave up, quit dialysis, became despondent and then died very quickly of kidney failure. They could see that I somehow had survived, and they wanted to know my secret. I said it was the support and spirit of my wife. That she would not allow me to give up and faithfully took me to every dialysis appointment. She not only took me, but then found something to do to wait around the five hours it took for each procedure. Without her, I would not be telling this story.

As I started the procedure, I talked to my wife about the need for the seemingly endless trips to this facility, every other day. She asked about the long-term prognosis, and I told her it did not look good. That I would need to get lucky to land a kidney. She told me we had to go through it if there was even a chance that it would prolong my life. For the next year and a half, I traveled an hour every other day to sit in a chair for 5 hours while they drained my blood, cleaned it, and then put it back in me. Then, my wife would pick me up and we would drive back to our house for the last hour. I originally had a portal in my chest that allowed the technician to connect directly into my bloodstream. They wanted me to go to a cardiologist who would connect an artery to a vein in my arm (called a fistula) that would make it easier to dialyze me.

I went to the cardiologist, who said it was a simple procedure that would require simple anesthesia. It could be done quickly, and it would be day surgery. I would be home by the afternoon. Things went smoothly for several months, but then during the preparation for dialysis by a newly trained nurse, she poked through the newly created fistula completely.

Dialysis requires highly specialized equipment and specially trained personnel. There was a pecking order with personnel in the facility. There was always a head nurse in overall charge, a nurse who was a specialist in poking veins, and usually a "newbie" who was learning the overall operation.

I have very skinny veins and at times the hospital phlebotomist would have to call in their version of "Davy Crockett" to get an IV installed. But the rupture of the vein not only precluded dialysis that day, but the clot also required a new procedure performed by the cardiologist. The penetration had caused a clot to form. The clot would have to be removed and I would need to have the "fistula" reinflated, and a shunt installed.

This procedure was done under a local anesthetic and went very well initially, but as they increased the pressure required to install the shunt, it became increasingly painful. I remember thinking what am I going to do if this went "on and on". The pressure increased while the doctor would say, "We're not there yet."

Eventually, it was installed successfully, and I went to dialysis the next day. I went back to every other day sitting in a chair for 5 hours, draining my blood to be cleaned and put back into me. A modern medicine miracle, since I remember a time when dialysis was something that was rarely allowed and required a committee to be involved to decide if you earned the right to have it at all.

Since I was healthier and could still walk and had all my appendages, I would occasionally be assigned to the "newbie". This went on for many months. But then the newbie nurse poked another hole completely through the shunted vein, and I had to go back to the emergency room to get the shunt repaired. I just chalked it all up to my usual bad luck. I was becoming very philosophical about my medical condition because it didn't seem to matter what I tried to do. Things just happened to me!

It is important to note that my life had degenerated into a thrice-weekly treatment that precluded any large travels to sites that were out of the area. However, I traveled to Idaho, Oregon, and north to Bellingham. Each travel was limited by local access to dialysis chairs which required tremendous planning by my wife. She had to make sure that the local dialysis center had openings and then inform my current dialysis center so they would send my data to the new center.

This was also in the middle of COVID, so I was usually isolated from the main group undergoing their regular dialysis sessions. There were dialysis cruises, but they were prohibitively expensive. My wife did manage to schedule three minor trips that were within car travel distance. One trip was almost 500 miles to Bend, Oregon.

I relished any variance in my routine, but it could be very difficult to deal with the new centers' rules and procedures.

I also struck a mentor relationship with one of the nurses who was struggling through a chemistry course. It had been years since I had taken organic chemistry, but I tried my best to help him. His professor had asked a very esoteric and difficult question. It took some serious study on my part, but I was able to help him. He was also the "Davy Crockett" of that facility and could always find my veins, while it could be troublesome for some of the nurses (I have very small veins).

It seemed as if dialysis would be endless. I would be sitting in a chair having my blood drained out of me, cleaned, and put back into me. I could see no way out. I could see my life-extending for years with every other day, poked in a vein and forced to sit and watch TV. I could not really venture more than I could drive or travel to anywhere that was beyond a dialysis appointment every other day.

Cruises or airplanes were out of the question without guaranteeing a dialysis chair during or at the end of any trip. My wife managed to get us as far as Northern Washington and Central Oregon. It took tremendous organizational skills to work that magic. To think of going further afield, like the East Coast, Mexico, or Hawaii was out of the question.

In order for us to travel at all, she had to find a dialysis center that had an opening. Then she had to contact that center and have our dialysis center request the use of the opening for a certain week and send the necessary documentation of my condition to the center with the opening. Then confirm with the staff at the center that I would be gone for that week. Then she would have to find lodging for us and contact our friends that we would be there for that week.

Also, she had to let our friends know that on certain days I would be unavailable due to five hours spent in a chair and she would have to stay in the vicinity to return me. This was a truly daunting effort since most centers did not have travelers at all, so they were unfamiliar with the process. Any gaps or slowness could jeopardize the entire effort.

Although I could observe my fellow dialysis patients during their treatments. They all looked grey and not healthy at all. Many had amputations or were in wheelchairs. It gave me an entirely new perception of how lucky I was to still be pink and able to walk to dialysis.

Up to now, I had been seeing what many people were dealing with in their lives, which gave me a new perspective on my own life. I appreciated what my life, wife, and family had given me. I started to wonder how I could give back hope. I decided to write a book concerning aspects of my new medically supported life. Thus, I wrote my first book, "Hospital Survival" to both get rid of the demons that the medical establishment created for me personally and also to discuss how any person needs to learn before they end up in a hospital.

As I stated before, it was the middle of COVID, so I got the vaccine as soon as possible. I also have received each new booster as it is developed. My wife had COVID twice, but each time isolated herself from me to ensure that I did not become exposed. She caught it from a trip she took without me. She went to Napa Valley and foolishly drank samples of wine at a tasting bar. Having been vaccinated and boosted, she thought that she was protected. She is still very protective of my health and isolated to avoid transferring the virus to me.

ANOTHER SURPRISE GIFT

I was resigned to go to dialysis forever when another bolt from the blue was received from the hospital. A new kidney was now available, and could I get to the hospital within the next three hours? My wife was finally taking some time for herself and had gone to play pickleball. I called the only other person who I knew to be home in the middle of the afternoon.

My mom came to my rescue, she was twenty miles away but arrived within minutes. We drove off quickly and luckily found my wife on the courts. She loaded me into her car, and we drove off to catch the nearest ferry. Luckily again, it was the middle of the day, so there were no lines for the ferry. As it was, I barely reached the hospital within three hours. I went directly to the transplant center to check in, while my wife parked our car.

I was checked in quickly and given a room. Almost immediately, I was informed by a transplant nurse that the doctor had a tough day and was very tired. Could we do the operation tomorrow? I thought of all the commotion I had caused and started to say something, but then I realized that the last thing I wanted was a tired surgeon trying to save my life. If they thought I and the kidney were safe to do tomorrow, far be it from me to suggest that I wasn't ecstatic with a new kidney.

The next morning, I was awakened at 5:00 AM to begin the preparations for the new kidney. I was introduced to the anesthesiologist, who spoke very broken English. I had no idea what nationality he was, and I really didn't care, as long as he did his job.

I have noticed that after more than 5 major surgeries, my previous steel trap memory is no longer there. I understand that is a common issue for patients who survive major surgeries. It is definitely very true because I now need to make notes about major appointments. I went to sleep and woke up in the afternoon. I had a scar on my side and a swollen belly.

But for once, the operation had gone like clockwork. I recovered quickly and left the hospital three days later in a wheelchair, my wife gently assisted me in getting into her car, and we drove home. I felt like a million bucks.

I no longer had to do dialysis, it was relatively painless as it healed, but I could use the bathroom whenever I needed. Because of the dialysis, my bladder had shrunk in size dramatically. I now need to use the bathroom at least three times a night. It's disruptive, but far better than spending hours in dialysis. I really don't mind.

I had one more issue. Before the operation, they had installed a shunt and catheterized me. They had long ago removed the catheter, but the shunt remained to be removed. Shunts sometimes get embedded in your tissues, which is what occurred in my case. They had to reach up my urethra and grab the shunt and pull it out. It sounds as pleasant as it actually was. I nearly passed out.

Since my last operation, I am now 4 years from even attending meetings in a hospital. I insist on meeting my doctors in Zoom meetings.

I still meet my liver doctor every six months. I see an endocrinologist every quarter (I am diabetic), meet my kidney doctor every six months, and the surgeon who performed the liver transplant once a year. They all require complete blood tests before their appointments. My wife is addicted to pickleball and travel. We have taken many cruises, now that I am free of dialysis, which I enjoy very much. I am addicted to tournament poker, which I usually win on cruises.

A NEW BEGINNING

I have been a storyteller my whole life. I can remember keeping my friends enthralled on the bus for the hour it took to get to grade school with tales of the power of dirty dishwater. Later in my first job as a chemist, I would make up stories of how the compounds I was making for the DIY industry were based upon their history and thus they became relatives of compounds that were based upon existing formulas.

When I became a manager and was responsible for writing major responses to our proposal on how we would fulfill a government contract, I would regale the Navy with stories of how we accomplished our portions of the contract. I always tried to make it both interesting and informative.

Although I have been officially declared disabled since my hip infection and subsequent surgeries, I have been unable to just idle away my time watching my grandchildren grow up and keeping my wife relatively happy. I have been restless to continue to try and be productive in my life. Granted that my wife comes first om everything, but I also help with grandchildren, and helping my 99-

year-old mother cope with injuries from a fall that have limited her capabilities but not her mind. I try to see her every day if I can, play some cribbage, talk politics, and discuss family issues as they arise. My wife is an avid pickleball player and goes to play sometimes two times a day. I do spend a lot of time thinking about issues and calling my friends to have debates. I started to write down my experiences in my first book "Hospital Survival" to help rid myself of the demons and scares created in my first five months of hospital living.

My second book detailed the changes I went through from my staid strait-laced high school years to my crazy persona during my college days. I was quite the rebel and suddenly discovered how wonderful girls were. I called it "Dorm Rats" since that was the term used at the time for denizens of the campus domiciles. I then took a hiatus as I recovered from my gallectomy, liver/kidney transplants, dialysis, and a newly discovered zest for life in my new world. After I was contacted by a publisher from Canada "Explora Books", I really got excited by my need to relate how I survived for all these years with my sense of humor still existing and my love for my wife still emanating from my soul.

My third book (Spirit Beach) was about a fictional professor growing up on a beach similar to the area where I grew up and is based upon the muse that helped me through my early youth and growth. It contains both facts and fiction about life on a beach in the Northwest of America.

EPILOGUE

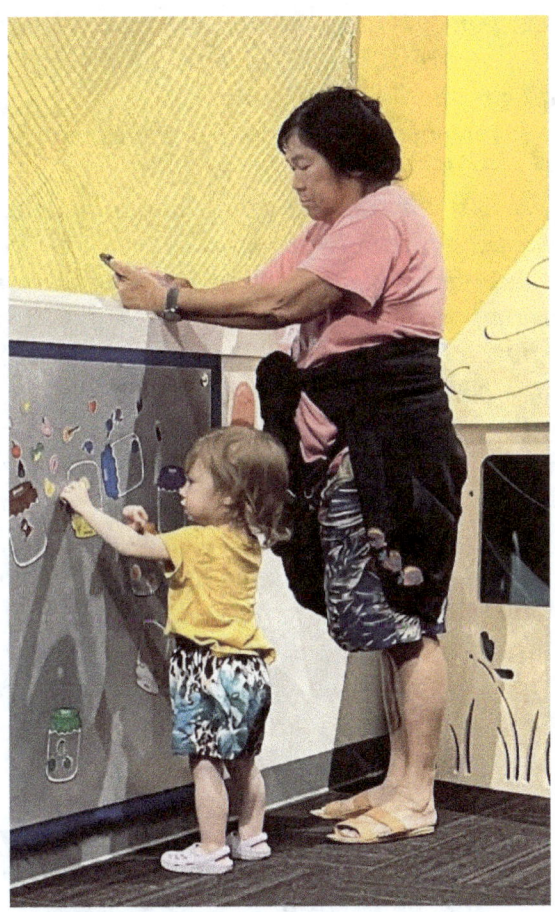

My wife & our youngest granddaughter

My wife is the true heroine of this story. Not only did she help keep me together to survive, but she put most of her life on hold as I recovered, while she continued to work until her school system allowed her an early out. As long as she would not work as a substitute teacher. She said "No problem"; a decision they later regretted when COVID hit and teachers were difficult to find.

I began to relate to the story of Job from the Old Testament. It seemed like every time I began to get lucky, something new would strike me that I and my loved ones would have to help me overcome. Thank God, they persevered, and I finally have got the point where I can relate the story calmly.

I will admit that my whole outlook on life has changed drastically. Earlier in my life, I was always driven to succeed. I loved challenges to me personally and professionally. I searched for approval from my bosses, my co-workers, and most of all my family. Since my exposure to death and my recovery; I am much more relaxed in all my behaviors. I appreciate my wife and friends every day.

Now, I use my story to "Wow" my new companions at dinner tables on cruises. Usually, the story is met with incredulity by the amazed people at the tables for lunch or dinner. After the discussion they say "Wow, your still alive and walking." Or "you're a miracle man". I usually respond with, "Yep, as long as it is flat and not too far, I am okay".

One individual went to great lengths to discuss my out of body experience when I died on the who interviewed survivors of death/near death experiences. She asked many detailed questions concerning what I saw and what I did during the experience and the reactions by the ICU personnel. My identification of a red shoe on the roof (There is one known by only a few nurses) and my feeling of omnipotence and ability to swirl the planets just by extending the thought got me some special attention in the hospital. The individual questioning me wanted to know if I had seen a white light or found a new belief. I disappointed her in my statements. I talked about my loss of a fear in death and my new ability to express my feelings. It was far more significant than that. It changed my whole life in ways that are difficult to cover.

I am much more considerate and loving than I ever was before. When I was a child, I would read encyclopedias for entertainment. I was always very competitive in life, debate, love and conversations. Partially because I grew up in a family and encouraged free thought and debate. I had an older brother who was very accomplished I sports, so I learned to compete with my mind. I was incorrigible in trying to one up anyone in work, play, or life.

Now I have changed considerably. Partly because I am handicapped and no longer have a career on which to compete. I help as much as I can. Enjoy my grandchildren and write some interesting books. I read a lot and watch too much TV. I cry at most tear-jerking movies, or heartful comments or stories.

During one conversation on the cruise ship, the person next to me was incredibly interested in my out of body experiences. Partially, because I did not make it seem like a big deal, just something that happened to me at the time. But I have changed dramatically from my former self in many ways; but I could see she was looking for more concrete religious changes and that didn't happen. I did not see God or sit by the throne; I just have newly found respect for others and my need to do things differently in my life.

At times, I give the impression of being an eternal optimist. That was not my original nature. If I give the impression that I overcame all my health issues, without any struggle, that is far from the truth. Many times, I was depressed. My foundation throughout all my struggles was always my wife and my family. There is absolutely no way I would have survived as a sane man, if it were not for their love and comfort. My discussions always give full credit for all their love and support. Otherwise, I would not be alive and writing it now.

APPENDIX I

Some insight from Wikipedia

The Liver

The liver is a major metabolic organ found only in vertebrate animals. It performs numerous essential biological functions, including the detoxification of the organism, the synthesis of proteins and biochemicals necessary for digestion and growth, carbohydrate metabolism, hormone production, and the decomposition of red blood cells.

The human liver is located in the right upper quadrant of the abdomen, below the diaphragm and mostly shielded by the lower right rib cage. It is a dark reddish-brown, wedge-shaped organ with two main lobes of unequal size and shape. The average adult human liver weighs approximately 1.5 kilograms (3.3 pounds) and has a width of about 15 centimeters (6 inches), though there is considerable size variation between individuals.

The liver is connected to two large blood vessels - the hepatic artery, which carries oxygen-rich blood from the aorta, and the portal vein, which carries blood rich in digested nutrients from the gastrointestinal tract, spleen, and pancreas. These blood vessels subdivide into small capillaries called liver sinusoids, which then lead to hepatic lobules.

Viewed from above, the liver is divided into a right and left lobe, separated by the falciform ligament. Viewed from below, it is divided into four lobes - left, right, caudate, and quadrate.

The liver produces bile, an alkaline fluid containing cholesterol and bile acids, which helps emulsify and break down dietary fat. The gallbladder, a small pouch under the right lobe of the liver, stores and concentrates the bile produced by the liver before it is excreted into the duodenum to aid digestion.

As of 2018, liver transplantation remains the only long-term treatment option for complete liver failure, as artificial livers have not yet been developed for sustained replacement.

Impressions of the liver

Several impressions on the surface of the liver accommodate the various adjacent structures and organs. Underneath the right lobe and to the right of the gallbladder fossa are two impressions, one behind the other and separated by a ridge. The one in front is a shallow colic impression, formed by the hepatic flexure and the one behind is a deeper renal impression accommodating part of the right kidney and part of the suprarenal gland.

The Liver - Functions and Diseases

The liver is a vital organ that supports almost every other system in the body, carrying out an estimated 500 separate functions. Some of the liver's key roles include:

Protein Metabolism: The liver is responsible for the synthesis and degradation of most plasma proteins, as well as a large portion of amino acid synthesis. It produces clotting factors and regulates red blood cell and platelet production.

Lipid Metabolism: The liver performs cholesterol synthesis, lipogenesis, and the production of triglycerides and lipoproteins. It also secretes bile needed for fat digestion and absorption of fat-soluble vitamins.

Detoxification: The liver breaks down and excretes many waste products and toxins, including bilirubin, ammonia, and various medications/drugs. It plays a key role in the body's defense against toxins.

Despite its impressive capabilities, the liver is prone to a number of diseases that can impair its critical functions. Some of the most common liver disorders include:

Non-Alcoholic Fatty Liver Disease: The accumulation of fat in the liver, affecting an estimated one-third of the global population.

Hepatic Encephalopathy: A condition caused by the buildup of toxins normally removed by the liver, which can lead to coma and death.

Budd-Chiari Syndrome: Blockage of the hepatic veins draining the liver, resulting in abdominal pain, fluid accumulation, and liver enlargement.

Jaundice: Characterized by yellowing of the skin and whites of the eyes due to increased bilirubin levels from impaired liver function.

Diagnosis of liver disease typically involves liver function tests, imaging studies, and sometimes a liver biopsy. For patients with irreversible liver failure, a liver transplant may be the only treatment option.

Understanding the diverse functions of the liver and the diseases that can impact it is crucial for maintaining overall health and well-being. This appendix provides an overview of this critical organ's key roles and associated pathologies.

APPENDIX II

Kidney Placement and Functions

Kidney Placement

Each human normally has two kidneys positioned on either side of the torso under the gastrointestinal tract and above the hips. The kidneys are located in the retroperitoneal space, nestled against the posterior abdominal wall.

Kidney Functions

The primary function of the kidney is to filter the blood and remove proteins, waste products, and other substances from the body. The kidney is composed of over a million nephrons, which are the functional units responsible for this filtration process.

When blood passes through the nephrons, waste products and excess water are filtered out, while vitamins, nutrients, and other essential molecules are returned to the bloodstream for continued use by the body. The filtered waste, known as urine, is then sent via the ureters to the bladder for eventual removal from the body.

In addition to filtration, the kidneys also play a critical role in:

- Maintaining fluid balance and blood pressure
- Regulating red blood cell production
- Activating vitamin D for calcium absorption
- Secreting hormones like renin to control blood pressure
- Any damage or impairment to the kidney's filtration and regulatory functions can allow dangerous levels of waste products to build up in the body, leading to serious health issues.

The performance of the kidneys is typically monitored by measuring creatinine levels in the blood. Elevated creatinine indicates decreased kidney function and the potential onset of kidney disease.

Kidney disease can be caused by a variety of factors, including diabetes, high blood pressure, infections, and exposure to toxins. Proper maintenance of kidney health is essential for overall bodily wellbeing.

APPENDIX III

Glossary

Acrylics	Acrylic resin is commonly used in latex paints as a binding agent.
Acupuncture	The traditional Chinese technique of inserting tiny needles along meridians believed to balance the "chi" or life force energy.
Albumin	A protein produced by the liver that helps regulate fluid levels and transport hormones and other molecules throughout the body.
Anesthetic	A substance used to block pain or induce sleep during a medical procedure.
Atrophy	The progressive deterioration or wasting away of muscle or nerve tissue.

Bilirubin	A compound that indicates how well the liver is breaking down old red blood cells.
CAT Scan	Computerized Axial Tomography, a scan that uses X-rays to create three-dimensional images of internal structures.
Chi	The Chinese concept of the body's vital life force energy flowing through specific meridians.
CMV Virus	Cytomegalovirus, a virus known to attack kidney structures in immunocompromised patients.
COBRA	The Consolidated Omnibus Budget Reconciliation Act, a federal program allowing terminated employees to continue their health insurance coverage.
COVID	A virus in the SARS family of coronaviruses.
Creatine	A compound produced naturally in the body that indicates kidney function by measuring protein filtration levels.
Cribbage	A card game played by 2-4 players, won by the first to reach 121 points through a series of dealing, playing, and showing phases.
Dialysis	A procedure that drains, filters, and returns cleaned blood to

	the body, often used to perform kidney functions.
DT	Delirious tremens, a life-threatening condition caused by withdrawal from addiction.
Endocrinologist	A healthcare professional who specializes in the effects of hormones on the body, especially for patients with diabetes.
Fistula	An abnormal connection between body parts, in dialysis a surgically created connection between an artery and vein to facilitate blood flow to the dialysis machine.
Glipizide	A medication that increases the body's natural production of insulin.
GS-4	An entry-level federal civil service position requiring a basic college degree.
Holistic	A discipline that treats the individual as a whole, rather than just individual organs or body parts.
Kahuna Anaana	A Hawaiian sorcerer believed to have the power to pray someone to their demise.
ICU	Intensive Care Unit.
Isocyanate	A family of highly reactive chemicals used in the production of foams.
Laparoscopy	Minimally invasive surgery using small incisions and a camera.
Lithotripsy	A non-invasive procedure to remove gallstones or kidney stones.

Mana	The Hawaiian concept of a spiritual, mystical power or force.
MASA	A membership program providing emergency ground or air transport to healthcare facilities.
MRI	Magnetic Resonance Imaging
Oceanography	The scientific study of the ocean, including biological, chemical, and physical aspects.
Oxycontin	A powerful opioid pain medication that was originally not listed as highly addictive.
Phlebotomist	A medical professional trained to draw blood or insert IVs.
Pseudomonas	A dangerous type of bacteria.
Recumbent	A bicycle that allows a reclining riding position, reducing stress on the hips.
RSV	Respiratory Syncytial Virus.
Septic/Septicemia	A life-threatening bacterial infection that has spread throughout the body.
Staph	Staphylococcus, a dangerous and difficult-to-treat bacterial infection.
Tacrolimus	An immune-suppressing medication that can cause bleeding problems.
Tamsulosin	A medication used to increase urine production.
Toluene	A substituted aromatic compound currently listed as potentially dangerous.
Trapeze	A device attached to a hospital bed to assist patients in transferring or changing positions.

Trichloroethylene	A chemical that may cause cancer and affect the liver and other body systems.
TSA	Transportation Security Administration.
UWMC	University of Washington Medical Center.
Urethra	The tube leading from the bladder that expels urine.
Vinyl-Acrylics	A cheaper resin used in paints compared to pure acrylics.

APPENDIX IV

Photos

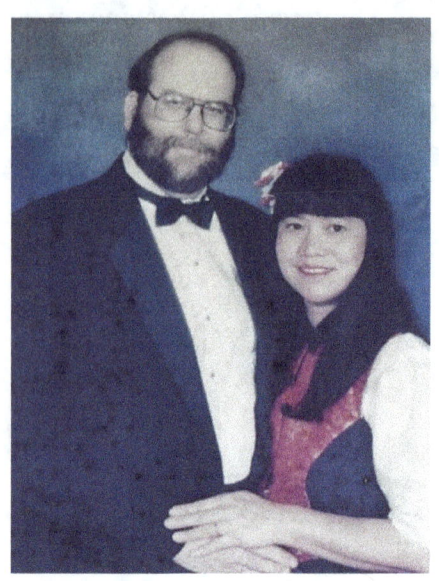

First Cruise Photo
(1989)

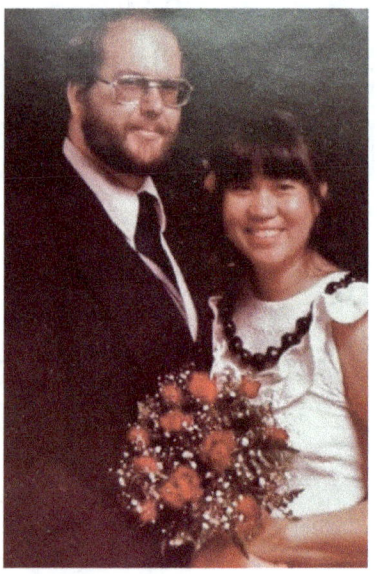

Wedding Photo
(1983)

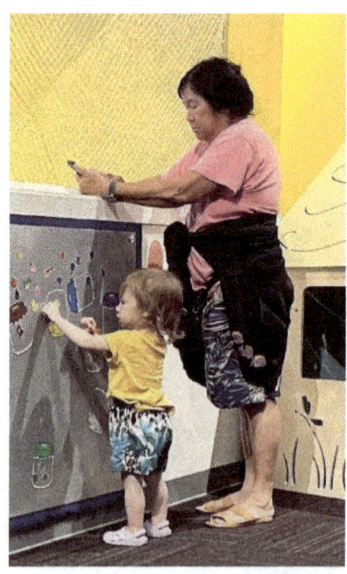

Granddaughter and My Wife
(2023)

www.ingramcontent.com/pod-product-compliance
Lightning Source LLC
Chambersburg PA
CBHW071215120626
46546CB00006B/2574